Essential Oils for

Psychedelic Therapy Support

An Introduction

to the

AromaGnosis Method

Florian Birkmayer, MD with Cathy Skipper

Table of Contents

Introduction

There has been a burgeoning interest in psychedelic therapy, but to my knowledge, there is virtually no information available on how to use aromatics, such as essential oils in this therapy. Both because of my longstanding interest in psychedelic therapy and years of experience using ketamine in combination with essential oils, as well as because of how my wife Cathy's and my approach of AromaGnosis has evolved, we felt a practical introductory book was urgently needed.

Aromas have been curiously overlooked as the powerful mind-altering molecules they are and for which plants evolved them. Now is the time to reclaim them as healing allies. We are also familiar with using aromatics with other psychedelic molecules and sacred plant medicines, so many of the approaches and insights discussed can be applied to those other forms of psychedelic therapies as they become more available.

This book is not in any way intended to provide any information or training on becoming a psychedelic therapist. While it may be informative to many different people, it is intended for therapists who are already trained in and have clinical experience with psychedelic therapy.

We discuss 5 essential oils in more detail in this book, so you can learn more about them and learn how to work with them. We consider these master allies for this work and a good starting point.

We also have developed a kit of these 5 oils, as well as a more in-depth online class. The details of both and more can be found in the Resources section at the end of the book.

At the core of this approach is our continued commitment to the archetype of the Wounded Healer. All of us, not just those of us that identify as healers, have to continuously commit to our own soul's healing journey so that we don't unconsciously project our inner wound onto the client, and thus keep them unconscious of their inner healer, and both them and ourselves trapped. At its core, this means accepting the reality of the unconscious. To be healthy means to continuously commit to getting our ego consciousness and our unconscious to cooperate. You can read more about the importance of the Wounded Healer at aromagnosis.com.

Psychedelic therapy and AromaGnosis can reawaken each of us to our inner healer and recommit us to an authentic life path. They can also both viscerally reconnect us to more of ourselves, our unconscious and to nature around us, which is part of our, or more accurately the transpersonal psyche. Through the sense of awe and bypassing the intellect, we can remember or realize we're part of something much bigger.

Healing this sense of connectedness is urgent in the world right now. Some thinkers, including Paul Levy, have talked about a hidden mental illness, like a mind-virus, that cuts us off from our own sacredness, each other, and nature and at the same time convinces us that there's nothing wrong with us in our cut-off-ness. Paul Levy calls this 'wetiko', a Native American term he borrowed.

Aromas and psychedelics are also important for the currently urgently needed healing of transgenerational traumas. Again, if you want to explore this topic more, please visit aromagnosis.com.

Aromas can enhance psychedelic therapy and also everyday personal growth.

We hope you find our approach helpful.

A Brief History of Psychedelic Therapy

Psychedelic therapy can be considered one of the oldest forms of therapy for soul healing and at the same time is now considered cutting edge in biomedical medicine after decades of being shunned. Using essential oils for psychedelic therapy support has not been discussed at all and as far as we can tell, we may be the first to use essential oils for psychedelic therapy support. However, we have heard from more and more people, including psychedelic therapists, who have started incorporating aromas into their practice, inspired by our approach. They have found it very rewarding and offering another, much sought for layer of benefit to psychedelic therapies. Aromatics have been used in several traditional societies for spiritual healing, both in combination with psychedelics and by themselves and this sacred heritage is being rediscovered and incorporated into present-day clinical practice.

A number of traditional indigenous societies, in almost all parts of the world, work with plant spirit medicines, which seems a more holistic and respectful term that psychedelic, for soul healing. (The only indigenous traditional society that doesn't use plant spirit medicines or psychedelic plants are the Intuit, which some speculate is due to the lack of psychoactive plants growing near the Artic.) In an oversimplified way, psychedelic therapy can be defined as the use of mind-altering or psychedelic (which literally means 'mind manifesting') plants and mushrooms for the purpose of healing a disease or imbalance that can manifest in the physical, emotional, mental, and spiritual bodies of an individual or group. The setting for this therapy can be individuals or groups. Most of the time, a shaman or similar person or group of persons guides the experience.

Starting with R. Gordon Wasson's 'discovery' of Maria Sabina, a Mazatec traditional healer who was working with psilocybin-containing mushrooms, in 1955, there has been growing interest in western societies in 'psychedelic therapy.' (However, we have to acknowledge the negative impact of R. Gordon Wasson and those who followed him on Maria Sabina's family and traditional Mazatec culture and healing practices. Similar negative impacts have been seen in other indigenous cultures when they are 'discovered' by 'westerners,' i.e. those living in a Euro-american cut-off culture.)

This is an oversimplified way of introducing the history of psychedelic therapy. Although there was interest in psychedelic molecules before then, such as anthropologists studying the use of peyote, the Nazis experimenting with mescaline on people incarcerated at Dachau and the discovery of LSD in 1943, to me these efforts were not with the intention of healing. Sandoz, the company for which Hoffman worked when he discovered LSD, used to give LSD away freely to any researcher or doctor who wanted to experiment with it, because they didn't know what healing potential it offered.

After a period of promising research in the 50's and early 60's (by Humphrey Osmond who coined the term 'psychedelic', and other people) which resulted in a significant amount of research, along with some truly revolting attempts to use these molecules for mind control (MK Ultra, Donald Ewen Cameron), the recreational use of psychedelics spread far and wide, the healing intentions and sacred focus were widely forgotten or obscured by sensationalist news stories and there was a widespread backlash against psychedelics. Their healing promise and the sacred tradition, along with the accumulated wisdom, was mostly forgotten.

Over the last 25 years, there has been a renaissance of official, academic research into psychedelic therapy, mostly focusing on psilocybin, MDMA, LSD and ketamine. Mainstream interest in and acceptance of these treatment approaches is spreading, as evidenced by more and more books and documentaries being released, more and more research centers being opened at various universities and more companies trying to figure out a way to profit from these sacred teachers.

At the same time, there has been a long and vibrant tradition of 'underground' psychedelic therapy, which has helped many people and kept the sacred traditions alive while gathering experiential wisdom. It is from this practice-based evidence that the importance of having a clear intention and having a pair of experienced sitters has been demonstrated, which has then also been reaffirmed in official studies.

With the current renaissance of psychedelic therapy research, which appears to be dominated by academic research centers, pharmaceutical and similar companies and treatment centers, it is important to remember the sacred legacy and the wisdom of indigenous traditions, that are, once again, at risk of being marginalized.

A Brief Introduction to Ketamine

Ketamine is currently (as of early 2024) the only FDA-approved medication that can be used for psychedelic therapy, although this is considered 'off-label.' Most of the research on ketamine has focused on outcomes, measures and rating scales, e.g. for depression, PTSD, etc., as well as the neurochemical and neurobiological changes that may contribute to ketamine's benefits, which include that it works on the NMDA receptor and appears to increase neuronal plasticity, which is the ability of neurons in the brain to form new connections and thus establish new patterns of thinking and behaving. We and a few others are also realizing the unique therapeutic potential of the psychedelic experience ketamine can offer.

The potential benefits of the psychedelic experience of ketamine, which some consider rather unique, have been mostly overlooked, although that is slowly changing. Both due to the psychedelic experience and neuronal plasticity effects. I think and researchers are beginning to show that ketamine and other psychedelics disrupt the Default Mode Network. I have started to suspect, and research demonstrates more and more, that the Default Mode Network, a widespread network of connections and centers in the human brain, is involved in most ongoing and long-standing emotionally distressing and dysfunctional patterns, including depression, anxiety, PTSD and trauma-spectrum disorders, addiction and other dysfunctional unconscious patterns. Many of these unconscious patterns are socially sanctioned, such as consumerism and ideological extremism, both of which are destroying nature and the unifying, mutually humanizing bonds of living with the awareness that we are an integral part of the larger than human ego world.

For a number of years, I have combined ketamine with essential oils, which in my experience can significantly enhance the healing process that ketamine offers. After briefly discussing how ketamine works, I will discuss a few essential oils that I have recently used with clients receiving ketamine and their benefits.

Ketamine is a dissociative anesthetic that has shown great promise as a novel treatment for depression (Fond et.al. 2014), PTSD and chronic pain. In my practice, I have also seen it provide benefit for OCD (Obsessive Compulsive Disorder) and there is early research to support this (Rodriguez et.al. 2013) and other conditions, such as autism-spectrum, that have not responded to more common medications. Ketamine has been FDA approved since the 1960s. Ketamine is most commonly given intramuscularly or intravenously, both in clinical practice and in studies, although there are other ways to deliver it, such an inhalation devices and lozenges. A recent survey of practitioners and review of the literature (Feifel et.al. 2020) indicated that ketamine has a low rate of serious side effects and that long-term treatment is reasonably safe.

A double case report I wrote on combining ketamine with essential oils was published in 2021. (Birkmayer 2021)

Combining aromas with other psychedelics, such as psilocybin, is also very interesting and offers potential for synergy and enhanced benefits of psychedelic therapy.

References

Birkmayer F. (2021). Using Essential Oils to Enhance the Effects of Ketamine Psychedelic Therapy in Obsessive Compulsive Disorder and Substance-Induced Psychosis (Two Case Reports). International Journal of Professional Holistic Aromatherapy. 9(4), p.15-22.

Feifel D, Dadiomov D, Lee KC, Safety of Repeated Administration of Parenteral Ketamine for Depression. *Pharmaceuticals* 2020, 13, 151; doi:10.3390/ph13070151

Fond, G.; Loundou, A.; Rabu, C.; Macgregor, A.; Lancon, C.; Brittner, M.; Micoulaud-Franchi, J.A.; Richieri, R.; Courtet, P.; Abbar, M.; et al. Ketamine administration in depressive disorders: A systematic review and meta-analysis. *Psychopharmacology* 2014, 231, 3663–3676, doi:10.1007/s00213-014-3664-5.

Rodriguez CI, et. Al. Randomized Controlled Crossover Trial of Ketamine in Obsessive-Compulsive Disorder: Proof-of-Concept. Neuropsychopharmacology (2013) 38, 2475–2483

The Unique Power of Scent in Ketamine Assisted Psychotherapy

Ketamine's dissociative effects mean that when it is given intramuscularly in sufficient dose, the person receiving it experiences dissociation from the body and most of the senses. (Note: This dissociation is quite different from the dissociation seen in PTSD and trauma-spectrum disorders.) It can be almost impossible to walk, write or talk and people report being disconnected from their senses, having difficulty with seeing, hearing and proprioception. People talk about leaving their bodies, not feeling their bodies or having no body awareness. However, the sense of scent seems to be uniquely enhanced through ketamine and people report profound experiences of synesthesia triggered by aromas. Some describe meeting the spirit of the plant through the aromatic molecules in an essential oil.

One aspect of how this may happen lies in neuroanatomy. All senses, except the sense of smell, are processed through an organ in the brainstem called the thalamus. It's like a mixing board for most sensory input. The reason you're not feeling the clothes on your skin right now is that the thalamus filters that out. The reason you can focus on a conversation with one person in a noisy setting is because the thalamus filters out the background sounds. Your eyes only really see what the thalamus tells them to see.

Scent is different. The olfactory nerves in our nose and olfactory bulb go directly into the limbic system, a network of brain areas involved with memory and emotion. Scent is the only sense that is not filtered by the thalamus. Furthermore, many aromatic molecules cross through the skin into the bloodstream and across the blood brain barrier into the brain. We have olfactory receptors in most parts of our brain and almost every organ in our body, we literally don't just smell with our noses but our entire body and brain. So even and especially during the ketamine experience, when a person is dissociated and all other sensory input is 'off-line', one can still smell and experience the effects of aromatic molecules.

Nevertheless, I feel that the above explanation is superficial. I suspect there are deeper reasons why aromas and ketamine have such unique synergy, beyond the anatomical explanation I offer above.

There are also powerful synergies of aromas with psilocybin and other classical psychedelics (mescaline, LSD, etc.), i.e. those molecules that exert their psychedelic effects through the type 2 serotonin receptor (often abbreviated as 5HT2A).

It's worth mentioning that MDMA (colloquially known as ecstasy or Molly) seems to dull the sense of smell and there are reports that people can't smell essential oils or other aromas while using MDMA. This raises the question of whether aromas should still be used with MDMA. While aromas have effects on the body and brain that are not dependent on conscious scent perception through the olfactory bulb on top of the nose, this dulling needs to be taken into consideration. It doesn't mean not to use aromas in this case, just to be aware of this phenomenon.

Using Essential Oils in Psychedelic Therapy

The most important consideration when using essential oils in combination with ketamine or other psychedelic therapy is that the essential oil is alive. Most essential oils are produced industrially, which destroys this aliveness and therefore these are useless as allies in this work. Ancient alchemists and Hildegard von Bingen called this aliveness 'viriditas' (https://www.healthyhildegard.com/hildegards-viriditas/), which translated means 'greenness' and refers to the aliveness of plants. To me, the essential oil of a plant is a manifestation of the soul of the plant. The essential oil is not a product or a tool, but a living teacher and ally or plant spirit medicine. You can recognize this aliveness by the deep soul-to-soul connection you can experience when smelling an alive oil. I've personally gotten goosebumps and even cried when first smelling some of these special oils. As I've deepened my relationship with some of them, by working with them for years, they have become long-term living allies that continue to teach and reveal. Alive essential oils are profoundly psychoactive, both in combination with ketamine and other psychedelic therapies and by themselves.

We only work with approximately two dozen oils, and recommend starting with even fewer, e.g. a handful, because it's much better to have a deep relationship with a few oils than a superficial relationship with hundreds. We need to have a deep relationship with each oil and aroma, a soul-to-soul connection, which is established by smelling them and working with them over time. Working with them includes smelling an oil as if in meditation and opening our awareness to their effects on our psyche, being attuned to the shifts in physical sensations, emotions, mental and spiritual patterns. This also means becoming familiar with the smell.

An oil may intuitively come to us and one way is that we suddenly smell its aroma, even if the actual oil isn't nearby. This has been called an olfactory hallucination, a term I really don't like. I prefer to think that, having established a soul-to-soul connection, this experience is the oil trying to get our attention, as if to say 'you or your client need me right now.' Only when we recognize the unique smell of each oil, the native language of aroma, can we know which oil is trying to get our attention.

How We Work with Essential Oils

We work with essential oils exclusively by letting the clients smell them. We put a drop on a scent strip (aka perfume test strip), which the client holds so they can bring it closer to their nose as needed. We usually work with one aroma at a time, sometimes two. We don't use diffusers since it is much more difficult to control the amount of scent in a room and to clear the scent in a room between clients. We also don't put our oils in products.

As discussed above, ketamine uniquely amplifies the sense of scent and the 'synesthesia' can be profound. With the help of ketamine one can really meet the spirit of the plant and the aromas are uniquely powerful in helping us transform. Often when clients struggle to go deep enough or confront Shadow issues, the ketamine opens the door, so to speak, and certain aromas do the actual work. For example, galbanum or labdanum are powerful for revealing Shadow issues and, if needed, rose attar can be added to provide comfort when the Shadow themes become intense.

Using essential oils in other forms of psychedelic therapy can also be very helpful, allowing the client to go deeper and transcend ego barriers, including fears, more easily. One of the most common experiences people who have undergone psychedelic therapy report is a sense of deep connectedness to nature and the world, for which the new word 'ecodelic' has been proposed. As I will elaborate further below, aromatic molecules are the Molecules of Connectedness and are uniquely suited to viscerally restore that sense of deep connectedness both by themselves and in combination with psychedelic therapy.

An Introduction to a Few Essential Oils

While there are many essential oils to choose from, I wanted to discuss five essential oils that we have found to be major allies for deep, inner work. As mentioned before these are profound both in psychedelic therapy and by themselves, without psychedelics.

Rose Attar (*Rosa damascena* in *Santalum album*) made from the precious, ancient roses cultivated in the Ganges valley near Kannauj, India. Rose petals (Rosa spp.) are hydro-distilled in copper stills and the distillate is captured in sandalwood essential oil. This is an ancient method for which Kannauj became famous centuries ago. This method is far superior in terms of capturing the soul of rose than other, more modern methods. Pure essential oil of rose is very rare and extremely expensive because it takes 18,000 pounds of rose petals to produce 1 quart (approximately 1 liter) of rose essential oil. This has led to widespread adulteration of rose essential oil. There is another modern method of extracting aromatic molecules from rose and other plants using organic solvents (such as toluene or hexane) to produce what are called 'absolutes.' These absolutes also contain other molecules found in roses that would not be part of the attar or essential oil and even after thorough washing, traces of the organic solvent remain. In our experience, absolutes of rose are usually dead and don't allow for the soul to soul communication between human and rose. Another modern method of extracting aromatic molecules uses carbon dioxide as a solvent and the resultant product is called a CO_2 extract. Again, in our experience, the harshness of this method, which requires the carbon dioxide to be cooled until it is liquid and put under very high-pressure results in aromatic products that are dead.

Small bottles of precious attars, especially rose attar, were treasured and passed from generation to generation as heirlooms. Rose attar has been mentioned in ayurvedic texts for centuries as a supreme

medicine. The sandalwood is like a bowl or cupped hands that holds
the aroma of the rose. Rose opens the heart. It's like a spiritual hug.
It's great for reconnecting to our soul, receiving compassion and
feeling self-compassion. I often use this first with clients new to
ketamine, if they are nervous about the effects of ketamine. I use it in
combination with other aromas, to provide a sense of being
enveloped by love and compassion as the client explores their shadow
issues more deeply during the ketamine experience.

Vetiver (Ruh Khus) (*Vetiveria zizanioides*), made from the roots of
an aromatic grass, is a superb grounding essential oil. This grass is
grown around the world to control soil erosion, which is symbolic of
its grounding properties. Grounding is the opposite of psychological
dissociation. For clients with severe PTSD, chronic dissociation is a
survival mechanism, but also a problem, because it means we can't
really heal. Dissociation prevents us from feeling and healing.
Dissociation is often described as feeling that everything is unreal or
under water, or that one feels like a head in the clouds or a head on a
stick, with no awareness of the body and the present moment. Vetiver
grounds us and reconnects us with our bodies, so we can feel, heal
and be here now. Vetiver can also provide grounding, if necessary,
during the more intense phases of ketamine therapy. Ruh Khus, a
Hindi term, refers to essential oil made from wild vetiver using the
traditional copper still, as opposed to from cultivated vetiver. This is a
pure essential oil, since vetiver yields a lot of essential oil and the attar
method is not needed.

Galbanum absolute is made from the resin of a Persian species of
fennel called *Ferula gummosa*. Galbanum resin is an ancient aromatic
that was already widely traded in the ancient world and is mentioned
in the old testament as one of the ingredients in Ketoret, the sacred
Jewish incense burned on the Sabbath. One of its purposes is to carry
the sacred energy of the sabbath into the other days of the week.
Galbanum is a great aroma for committing to change and a new path,
e.g. for helping clients with addiction commit to sobriety. It helps us

to stop delaying and waiting around and take action and commit to
the path ahead. 'The time is now,' it seems to say. In combination
with ketamine, it appears to help commit to the changes the
neuroplasticity of ketamine offers, but which require changes in
behavior and thought patterns. It is also powerful in bringing up
Shadow issues and allowing the client to go more deeply into the
ketamine experience to retrieve insights that are ready to be released
from the unconscious into consciousness, but that the ego may be
resisting out of fear of change.

Labdanum (*Cistus ladanifer*) is probably the most sacred aroma of the
ancient Egyptians who used a number of sacred scents as
sophisticated spiritual technology. Labdanum is the resin produced by
a species of cistus bush that grows widely in Mediterranean areas. One
of the scepters of Osiris is a labdanum resin collecting tool (often
mistakenly called a flail) and it was central to his archetype and myth,
which involves death, dismemberment and resurrection as well as
being able to travel into the unseen realms. We call it the Master of
Shadows, because it brings Shadow issues to the surface like nothing
else. When someone needs to and is ready to go deeper, to reveal
buried and forgotten traumas, labdanum takes you there.

Helichrysum (*Helichrysum italicum*) essential oil is made from a
Mediterranean shrub that is also called immortelle or everlasting,
because its flowers appear not to wilt. Helichrysum is great for
releasing and healing childhood trauma. It allows us to cry long-
suppressed tears and facilitates deep release coupled with a feeling
self-compassion. You can finally allow yourself to feel without
judgement. It also reminds you that it is much healthier to allow these
deeply repressed feelings to surface than to be continually running
from them. Helichrysum goes to the core, it doesn't beat about the
bush. In the context of ketamine, it's great for those who lack self-
compassion and need to cry the tears they have never allowed to
come up.

A Framework for Working with the Unconscious in Psychedelic Therapy

Another important aspect when working with the psyche is to have a good framework or roadmap for the unconscious. In brief, I find certain aspects of Jung's model (i.e. the alchemical stages) quite helpful for navigating the unconscious realms and being able to tolerate in ourselves and in our clients the challenging emotions that come up when we face the unconscious, heal, release traumas and individuate. You can read more about the alchemical stages in our blog post: https://aromagnosis.com/hello-world-2/

In my experience, most conventional psychiatric medication management is countertransference, i.e. the prescriber is asking the client to take a medication because of their own anxieties about the client and this sends the implicit message that challenging emotions should be covered up. Instead, if we are able to recognize and behold the challenging emotions related to personal transformation, we can allow the natural processes of the psyche to heal and reconnect us.

Alchemists were both the source of Jung's model of the psyche and in their own right explorers of the unconscious realms and also distilled some of the first essential oils. To me it's beautiful and deeply synchronistic to bring back together these two aspects of the alchemical tradition for healing.

A Holistic Model of the Human Psyche

Psychedelic therapy and deep work with the unconscious requires us to have a holistic model, that includes not just the client, but ourselves as practitioners, too. Otherwise it is easy to become overwhelmed by ego fears or to be taken over by the unconscious. In either case, we are not fully present. We need a way for the ego and the unconscious to learn to communicate and collaborate respectfully, in partnership, without either dominating or taking over.

There are many stages to advancing scientific knowledge. The nowadays much-touted 'evidence-base' and 'controlled studies' are only one step in establishing and advancing knowledge. Studies can only confirm or invalidate theories of an already existing model. The much earlier and much more important stage of research is to come up with new models. It is only when we come up with new models that we contribute to what Thomas Kuhn in "The Structure of Scientific Revolutions" (Kuhn, 1970) called a paradigm shift. This phrase has been tossed about and misused a lot recently.

This section is an attempt to sketch out a new model of holism based on the idea that aromas touch and reconnect us on multiple levels, from the molecule to the ecosystem. In a time when human beings' disconnection from Nature and the Collective Unconscious and the cult of the supremacy of the individual ego are destroying the environment and also the better angels of our human nature, we are being called to re-member, re-collect and re-connect ourselves as part of a bigger living being, called by many names, such as Mother Nature, Gaia and the Dark Goddess.

The role of aroma in shaping humans, again from the molecular to the cultural level, has been discussed in a piecemeal manner. What has been lacking is a truly holistic view. In behavioral sciences the term bio-psycho-social was coined almost 50 years ago. It went from an inspiring attempt at making behavioral health more holistic to an empty buzz-phrase that has been much abused. Holistic must not suffer the same fate. If we want to be holistic, we need to consider how to reconnect all levels of the psyche. The psyche isn't just a part of the physical body. The physical body is just one layer of the psyche.

If we want to be holistic, we also have to let go of an entire world view of pathology, which perceives that there are only identifiable diseases, often permanent and incurable. We also have to go beyond the idea that healing involves restoring some sort of equilibrium or a restoration of an earlier or imagined state of wellbeing or at least, and frankly most commonly, symptom relief without addressing the underlying problems.

Biomedical or 'western' medicine, and especially mental health care, lacks a positive definition of health. It only has a negative definition of health, meaning that health is merely the absence of disease. There are many 'diseases' described in the DSM-V (the Diagnostic and Statistical Manual, 5th edition, which lists the commonly accepted psychiatric diagnoses), but there's no definition of what is means to be healthy. One gift from Jung is a positive definition of health, which is that each of our lives gives us the opportunity to individuate, that is to discover our unique personal myth. This positive definition of health offers a road map or something to aim towards or to at least be open to.

We need to realize, instead of only focusing on symptoms and diseases, that each experience in life, especially challenging experiences, can be transformed into steppingstones for growth. "We become enlightened not by imagining figures of light," as Jung said, "but by making the darkness conscious." (Jung, 1945) Through these experiences we have the opportunity to grow, to understand ourselves better by establishing a respectful dialog with the unconscious and to reconnect with the seen and unseen dimensions of Nature. Aromas are the new royal road to the unconscious, and they are powerful allies in this holistic healing path.

Our Wound—for we are all Wounded Healers—reveals to us our personal myth. (Levy 2019) Our personal myth becomes our medicine for ourselves and to the world. Our true holistic healing is to reawaken to our personal myth. We have developed protocols to help people discover their personal myth, which combine aromas (by inhalation only) with drumming and guided meditation/journeying. Using aromas with ketamine can also open the doors to the unconscious that allow clients to discover and learn to embody their personal myth. When working with the psyche it is of utmost importance to have a roadmap or framework for opening our awareness to these parts.

References
Jung, C. G. "The Philosophical Tree" in Collected Works Vol. 13: Alchemical Studies, Bollingen, para. 335, 1945
Kuhn, T. „The Structure of Scientific Revolutions" University of Chicago Press; 2nd edition; 1970
Levy, P. "We are all Wounded Healers"
https://www.awakeninthedream.com/articles/we-are-all-wounded-healers, accessed 9/1/2019

The Concentric Circles: A Framework for Working with the Psyche

Inspired by Jung and indigenous philosophies, we have developed a framework or terrain map for working with aromas (be they essential oils, hydrosols or other natural aromas) holistically, either by themselves or in combination with psychedelic therapy.

The biggest trap in holistic healing and especially psychedelic therapy is to be trapped by the intellect. There's a big difference between thinking about an issue and working on an issue using our entire being. Working on our own Wounded Healer's journey is a prerequisite for being able to hold the space and create a sacred healing space when working with clients in this way. The Wounded Healer's journey is ongoing. As Jung's closest collaborator Marie-Louise von Franz said, "The Wounded Healer is THE archetype of the Self." The Wounded Healer's journey is the ongoing journey of Individuation through discovering and embodying our personal myth.

In order to be on the Wounded Healer's journey and to truly holistically work with the unconscious, using aromas as well as psychedelic therapy, we need to be aware of our physical bodies, our emotional bodies, our mental bodies, our spiritual bodies, our connection to the layers of the Collective Unconscious, and to catch glimpses of the Self, that encompasses all these layers (see figure 1 below). This is not intellectual awareness, but rather what I like to call 'heart awareness.' This is the awareness that has been referred to by various names such as 'the Observer' in several meditation traditions. Others call it the Witness. It is only with our open heart that we can truly perceive.

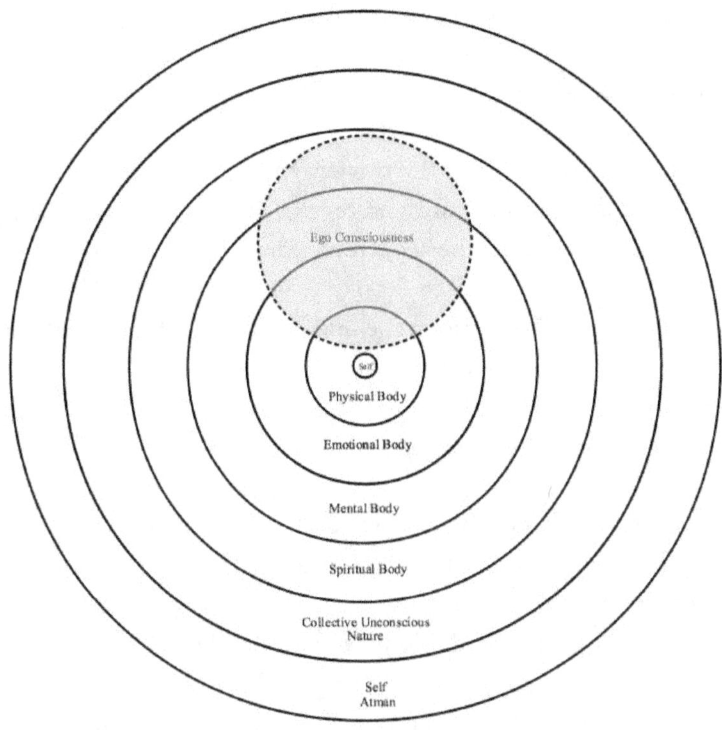

Figure 1: Anatomy of the Psyche: The Concentric Circles by Florian Birkmayer, MD

Figure 1 is a diagram adapted from Jung and other traditions. It is in the shape of a circle because, according to Jung, circles and mandalas are symbols of wholeness. Its purpose is to provide a map of the realms of the psyche so that we can assess what is happening in each 'layer.' Otherwise it's easy to confuse layers, e.g. a lot of people confuse feelings and thoughts. Furthermore, by remembering the Concentric Circles, we don't forget about and skip layers.

The smaller dashed, grey circle represents the ego. The ego contains our conscious awareness, also called **ego consciousness**. The reason I made it grey in this diagram is because one of the main tricks the ego plays on us is to convince us it is all there is. It creates a grey fog of separateness. In Jung's view the ego is really an epiphenomenon that arises out of the unconscious and returns to it. If you think your ego is stable and continuous, I have a simple question: Where does your ego go when you are sleeping?

There's a Buddhist story about a wave in the ocean that approaches the shore and as the wave curls and breaks, many little droplets briefly break off and fly through the air before rapidly returning to the ocean. For those brief moments, each droplet yells "I'm an individual." That droplet is the ego. The ocean in the unconscious, both personal and collective. The unstable, ever-shifting nature of the ego is represented in the Concentric Circles diagram by the dashes that form the circumference of the grey circle.

The ego covers a part of the physical body. Our ego individuality is strongly attached to our body. "I'm this body." Would there be an ego without the body? However, there are many unconscious ongoing processes in the body that don't depend on the ego. Your ego doesn't have to tell your heart to beat, your lungs to breathe, your guts and associated organs to digest, your tissues to grow, your physical wounds to heal. The ego circle doesn't just occupy part of the physical body layer because of course our ego awareness isn't just body awareness.

The ego also covers part of the emotional body, since we identify with our emotions. We have emotions that we are conscious of and we often project our unconscious emotions onto others.

The ego also covers part of the mental body. Descartes's famous "I think therefore I am." succinctly summarizes how our sense of ego is rooted in our mind.

The ego touches or includes a part of the spiritual body in those of us who know there are spiritual dimensions to our being. It may not, in those that don't think so, but it doesn't mean the spiritual realm doesn't exist or isn't important.

Now that we've briefly described the ego, let's look at the anatomy of the entire psyche, represented by the concentric circles.

At the center of the larger, concentric circles, which represent the totality of the psyche is a small circle labeled Self. This is our core sense of existence. Our essence. Our star. We will discuss this in more detail shortly.

The second smallest layer, represented by a circle in the diagram represents our **physical body**, which our human sense of self is usually centered and grounded in. Our sense of our body is very dense, but it is nevertheless a part of the psyche, although it has often been considered separate. It is more or less fixed and unchanging. I can't just change bodies. It is 'stuck' in the present moment, i.e. I identify with my body at the present moment, not a year ago or 30 years ago or 10 years from now. It feels solid and a very core part of our sense of self. Even though it may not be our complete sense of ego, for most people, our ego is inextricably linked to our physical body.

The next layer is the **emotional body** or emotional field. This represents all the emotions we have felt, are feeling, may still feel and are capable of feeling. Emotions are feeling states and often contrasted with thoughts. In several spiritual traditions, the emotional body is described as an invisible field around our physical body, that is less dense that the physical body, but shares some attributes. Even if this particular description doesn't make sense to some, our sense of self consists in no small part of the emotions we feel. "I" feel an emotion. With empathy we can feel another's emotion. Emotional bodies are less dense and more fluid and can resonate with other emotions around. When leading meditations, I always say that you can imagine your emotional body in any way that makes sense to your awareness.

In general, our feelings have no historicity, we identify with the feelings what we feel at that moment (although we can recall how we may have felt in the past), just as our sense of our body is of our body in the moment. Laughing is different than remembering the last time we laughed.

My sense of my body is that of a middle-aged man. I don't think my body that I identify with is the body I had when I was 16. It's very similar with our feelings. I identify with what I'm feeling now and not with what I'm not feeling or never felt. Furthermore, I project my unconscious feelings onto others. Projection is one of the core functions or tricks of the ego. We all project. What is inside the grey circle are 'my' emotions, that is the emotions I identify with and am willing to own. What is in the unconscious emotional layer of my psyche, are still my emotions, but I am unconscious of them, I don't own them, so my ego either represses them or projects onto other people. One of the most important political and spiritual things we can do is reel in our projections and thus become aware of them.

Of course, our emotions change much more quickly than our physical body. In dissociation, one could say that the person is cut off from their sense of feeling, i.e. their ego has shrunk away from the emotional body. In extreme cases of dissociation, such as fugue states and depersonalization/derealization, the traumatized ego has also withdrawn from the physical body. (We interestingly also see this in rare neurological conditions, e.g. hemi-lateral neglect after a stroke in certain areas of the brain, where a person no longer identifies with the side of the body affected by the stroke. The ego's attempts to make sense of this are fascinating. In medical school I saw a hospitalized patient with hemi-lateral neglect who, when asked who the arm he no longer identified himself with belonged to said, 'the nurse.' I saw another patient who, when encountering his neglected hand with his still non-neglected hand, would shake it and introduce himself, saying "Hello, my name is …")

The next layer is the **mental body** or mental field. You could imagine it, as many do, as an invisible field larger than the emotional and physical bodies. I find it helpful to think of it like a river of thoughts and we can either be swept along by our thoughts, which seems to be default state for most of us, most of the time, or we can cultivate awareness, e.g. through meditation, which is like sitting by the riverbank watching the thoughts go by. Aromas can help us gain this perspective of observing our thoughts without being swept away by them. Of course, we identify with our thoughts. The trick the ego plays on us is to convince us it is all there is and with this comes an overreliance and overvaluing of the mind and intellect at the expense of the other parts of the psyche and their combined wisdoms, which are much greater. The unconscious layer of thoughts are all the things we think, that we don't even know we think. This is where propaganda, advertising and other forms of manipulation occur. This is the realm of memes and thought viruses. We are also unconscious of the ruts our thoughts are in and with aromas, we can allow our thoughts to get out of these ruts. The overidentification of ego with thought has led to the cut-off-ness from our own souls, others and Nature that is the fundamental problem of modern humanity. When French philosopher Renee Descartes said "I think therefore I am," which is really one of the origin points of this overidentification, it's as if he cast a terrible curse. Through aromas and other methods, we can transcend this limited identification of ourselves with ego mind and reconnect to our souls and Nature all around us.

The next layer is the **spiritual body**. This is the realm of our inner unconscious masculine and feminine. We may identify with one and keep the other in the Shadow, i.e. the unconscious parts of the concentric circles outside the ego. Jung called the part in the shadow Anima (in men) or Animus (in women). While the Shadow is everything in the concentric circles outside the ego, it can also be personified. It can personify in each layer in each body. It could be a dream and thus in the mental and emotional realms. It could be a shadow projection onto a person in everyday life.

The next layer is really much deeper and more multilayered than can be represented in this diagram. It has been labeled the **Collective Unconscious**. Our ego doesn't touch it, even though the ego arises from there, the way a tree grows out of the soil or the droplet arises from the wave in the Buddhist story above, because it is completely unconscious. Another name for it is the Transpersonal Realm. Through aromas we can develop a respectful way of communicating with the realms of the Collective Unconscious. Nature is already doing this through the aromatic molecules of connectedness produced by plants and in many other ways. Of course, there are the realms of the ancestors in the Collective Unconscious and reconnecting with our ancestors is fundamental to restoring right relationship within ourselves and with Nature around us. The Collective also contains our family, our friends, our community, plants and animals and their relatedness to us. They are not just material beings around us, but we all arise out of and are deeply embedded in the Collective Unconscious. A mere ring of a circle in our diagram in no way adequately represents the multidimensionality of the Collective Unconscious. It is important to remember that the ego and the physical body as well as the other layers of the individual, as well as every material being and thing in the world, arise out of the collective unconscious, like a tree growing out of the soil.

The outermost layer is the **Self**, with a capital S, also known as Atman. The World Soul. The Unus Mundus (a Latin phrase that means 'One with the world' used by alchemists), when we identify with a larger awareness than our ego awareness. As we work on ourselves and catch glimpses of this Self, we develop our Personal Myth. This Self is really the same as the tiny Self at the center of the circle. It is a fractal.

The Molecules of Connectedness

"When we change 'I' to 'We', even Illness becomes Wellness." – Malcolm X

Aromas can touch us on and reconnect us with all our bodies. What does it mean to touch and to be touched? To us humans, the obvious answer is skin to skin contact. But what if you are a sessile being, for example a tree? How do you touch then? If the molecules that constitute our skin are part of us, are the aromatic molecules we emit part of us? Human lovers communicate deeply and desire through their mutual smells. Do trees touch each other and us through the volatile aromatic molecules they release into the air we all share?

When we are touched by an aromatic molecule, the molecule literally binds to one or more specific receptors in our body. Not just in our nose. We have olfactory receptors, of different subtypes, in virtually every tissue of our body. We don't just smell with our nose, we smell with every organ, with our skin, with our kidney, with our heart. This is one way aromas touch our physical body.

There are over six hundred genes in the human genome that encode olfactory receptors. And that is just the family of Olfactory Receptors (OR). There is another entire family of receptors called Transient Receptor Potential Channels (TRPC), which encode the feeling of coolness of mint and apparent heat of capsaicin and many other, as yet to be discovered, sensations. This is another way aromas touch our physical body and at the same time our mental body by inspiring us to come up with models and evidence, e.g. research on receptors.

If you think of each olfactory receptor as the letter of an imaginary alphabet, imagine what complex poetry/'words'/ideas/archetypes you could form with such an alphabet. Our English alphabet pales by comparison. We have, most of us, become completely unconscious of smell. We've lost our instinct. Yes, some may eloquently talk about beautiful aromas, essential oils or perfumes, but that is an intellectual construct, using language. What if we were still native speakers in the language of scent? This would mean remembering aromas don't just touch us intellectually, but emotionally and spiritually.

Why do we even have a sense of smell? Why do we have all these olfactory receptors? Since I was in medical school, I kept asking 'Why do we have dopamine as neurotransmitter?' Why this molecule and not another instead? Dopamine is not a very 'sensible' molecule to use as a neurotransmitter in a long-living human brain, since it forms a toxic breakdown product that accumulates in the brain. Why then use this molecule?

I came to realize that the reason we have dopamine and serotonin in our brains is that we inherited them from plants. Plants evolved dopamine and serotonin and the molecular machinery to make them millions of years before we ever walked the earth. In the same way that plants co-evolved with pollinators (e.g. bees) and developed aromatic molecules to influence the behavior of these pollinators, I believe that dopamine is there so that plants can influence our behavior—along with many other molecules, including aromatic molecules.

For example, all 'drugs of abuse' such as morphine, cocaine, are molecules that plants make and that increase dopamine in our brains. While they were in natural concentrations in plants and plant materials, they served a natural purpose, including healing, but then of course humans extracted and concentrated them and caused a disruption in the natural balance, that has had a profound impact on human history through addiction and other issues. In the same vein, we could ask 'Why do we have olfactory receptors?' Again, I think plants wanted to make sure that they could communicate with us.

Aromatic molecules touch us at the smallest material level, the closest distance. I touch and I am touched. This is not just a metaphor.

In my work with people with addiction issues I learned that what underlies most addiction is psychological trauma. This includes not just abuse but neglect, not just personal but collective, not just the experiencer, but historical/inherited/epigenetic trauma. There are layers and layers of trauma, some of which we may be conscious of, but most layers of which are in our unconscious.

And of course, there is the inescapable trauma of the world, as the environment is being destroyed by human activity and neglect. The word trauma comes from the Greek and means cut or wound. Trauma doesn't just hurt the body and the soul, but it also cuts us off from our spirituality, and our meaningful connections to the beings around us. Trauma literally cuts us off from our rich, natural environment and leaves us in a void, be it in the meaningless wasteland of cities and endless suburbs, nature cut apart, or in the prison of our suffering minds, addicted, seeking redemption, that bliss that we all remember, the Garden of Eden of connectedness.

It seems that history is just an endless story of trauma after trauma. The oldest stories we have, e.g. The Book of Job or the Epic of Gilgamesh, are full of trauma. I think we humans evolved storytelling as a way of trying to heal from and integrate trauma.

So much for a brief outline of trauma, being cut-off, being disconnected from nature and dissociated from Self. Now let's look at aromatic molecules and why they seem so perfect for healing trauma. They are perfect, because they are the Molecules of Connectedness.

Aromatic molecules travel through the air that connects all living beings. In many spiritual traditions the word for spirit is same as the word for breath and air, e.g. *pneuma* in ancient Greek, *ruach* in Hebrew, etc. Even the English word *awe* carries this between its meaning and its sound--that is we make a slow, open-mouthed exhale, a spirited breath.

The first thing we do when we are born is that we inhale and the last thing we do as we die is exhale. The air we exhale is inhaled by others. Plants turn our exhaled carbon dioxide into oxygen which we in turn need to breathe. We are connected to all living things through the air we breathe.

The air is between and within all of us and forms a giant presence around and within us all, a great spirit that we are all part of. If spirit is air, then the volatile aromatic molecules could be seen as the 'neurotransmitters' of this spirit, or conduits, messengers within the spirit realm. In Alchemy this is Mercurius, the ever-changing messenger, reconciler of opposites, as hard to capture as a scent or the wind. Through their very nature, aromatic molecules reconnect us.

The opposite of addiction is connection. How perfectly we are touched and healed by these Molecules of Connectedness to heal the trauma that has cut us off.

Aromas touch all layers of the concentric circles, conscious and unconscious. We can't not be touched; we can't switch off the effect.

A lot of research and clinical use of aromatherapy focuses on the physical body, including many studies on wound healing and antimicrobial activity. There are countless examples.

There is some research on the emotional effects, i.e. how aromas touch the emotional body although it is mostly focused on relief of specific symptoms or diagnoses. Aromas can also be used to explore unconscious and hidden emotions. Certain essential oils reliably allow people to become aware of unconscious emotions, including hidden aspects of trauma and by beholding and feeling these emotions, transform them. "To feel is to heal." Aromas that are masters of this are rose attar *(Rosa damascena* in *Santalum album)*, wild vetiver (*Vetiveria zizanioides)* and Labdanum (*Cistus ladanifer)*, which we refer to as the Master of Shadows.

On the emotional level aromatic molecules touch us in multiple ways. They evoke certain emotions and can rapidly shift our emotional state. In addition, they can highlight emotional blockages within us and bring emotions out of the shadow of our unconscious. When we are unconscious of certain feelings, we project them outwards onto others and Jung himself said that "the most important political and spiritual work we can do is to reel in our projections."

In the mental bodies, aromatic molecules inspire and generate much research, a mental venture, in addition to the forming of schools and organizations. Aromas have had a profound cultural impact. For example, the Dutch got to occupy the Banda islands in the south Pacific, the original source of nutmeg, by swapping it with the British for an island that was much less important at the time, called Manhattan. Nutmeg, a spice cherished for just its aroma, had a profound influence on world history. What if the British didn't colonize Manhattan and New York? The trade in coffee and other aromatic molecules continues to perpetuate colonialism. Human beings can clearly be mentally possessed by aromas and they have shaped history.

On the other hand, aromas can lead to mutual recognition, an 'I am thou,' which is part of the awareness of connectedness. Aromas have their own mental bodies, one of the layers of their wisdoms.

In the spiritual bodies, aromas have long been used as ceremonial incense, to pray, to connect, for meditation, for ritual, for invoking the ancestors and reliably give us that sense of awe. Blue Lotus was central to the spiritual practices of the Ancient Egyptians, along with countless perfumes and many still well-known aromatic substances were already made by them millenia ago.

Aromas touch the Collective Unconscious, for example as shown in the history and practices mentioned above. Aromas play an important role in cultures around the world, such as attars in ancient India and Persia and countless other examples.

In this collective realm, ancestral worship, practiced by all traditional cultures around the world, involves aromas, including marigold, tuberose and a variety of incenses. It is said that the dead eat with their sense of smell. Aromas reconnect the living and the dead and without this connection we cannot be truly holistically healed.

We can also use this model, the Concentric Circles, to explore how one essential oil touches us on all these levels. Rosemary (*Rosmarinus officinalis*) has a wide range of physical uses, including clearing the respiratory tract. On an emotional level is can raise our mood and be uplifting and energizing. On a mental level is has long been known to help memory, which has also been supported by research. On a spiritual level, it brings grace to our lives. As its name implies, the dew (ros) of the sea (marinus) rises from the surf like Venus, it reawakens us to spirit in matter, grace in suffering and was highly revered by the alchemists since it represented the approaching conjunction, the goal of the alchemical process. It was the 16th century alchemist Raymond Llull who first distilled rosemary essential oil. On the collective level, there is much lore about and recipes with rosemary in different cultures, from grief to love.

In summary, aromas reconnect us. They are 'ecodelic.' Aromatic molecules are the Molecules of Connectedness, and we all deserve to feel reconnected.

Connecting with an Essential Oil

Give yourself the space and time to do this exercise correctly, somewhere where you are comfortable and won't be interrupted.

Pick an essential oil without looking at what it is, and even if you recognize its smell, don't start thinking about its properties or indications. This is not the aim. Hold the bottle a few inches from your nose and allow the aromatic molecules to enter you. Better yet, put a drop of the oil on a scent strip and hold the strip under your nose.

Do not think about what the oil is or what constituents are in it or if you can name the scent.

Switch off your analytical, chatty brain. Spend a few minutes following your breath. As you do so, encourage your breathing to relax and deepen. Sink into your body and allow your consciousness to be aware of how the aromatic molecules feel in your body.

Remember when smelling an oil, we must feel it not think it!!

Where can you feel the aroma? What type of feeling is it? What movement is it making? Does it stay in one part of the body or does it move around, etc.? Just keep feeling with your body.

Notice if the soul of the plant in the aroma comes across a blockage or stagnation or resistance in the body. If it does, just witness it. Plants are very good at letting us know where energy is not flowing correctly. This is information that can help you understand what is going on for you.

Apart from the physical sensation that you feel when communing with plant aromas, you may experience emotions coming up. Again, just allow what wants to reveal itself to do so. There is nothing to do, nothing to change, just allow and witness. By acknowledging an emotion or feeling, it comes into consciousness and can heal.

Remember, *'to feel is to heal!'*

'Direct depth perception of a plant or any other phenomenon in nature will always reveal dimensions to its being that science can never see because these dimensions are invisible to the linear mode of consciousness' from "The Lost Language of Plants" by Stephen Buhner

A Guided Holistic Meditation Practice using Essential Oils and the Concentric Circles

Here's a practical way to use the concentric circles to really connect with an essential oil and to have it reveal to us what is going on in our psyche (remember the physical body is just one layer of the psyche). You should do this practice by yourself and then guide your clients through it and then encourage your client to practice it on their own. *It is helpful to practice this before giving a client ketamine or introducing aromas to the ketamine or other psychedelic therapy sessions.* Aromatic allies could be used without this model, but without this framework, it is easy to get lost in the unconscious realms that ketamine and other psychedelics take us into.

You can do this practice as a meditation and you can also do it while journaling. When you write in your journal use the Concentric Circles as a guide.

At first, it's best to start with single essential oils for this practice and see how one essential oil touches you on all these levels.

When you have some practice and experience, you could use two or more essential oils. For example, you can use a different oil for each body in the concentric circles. Try different ways. We strongly encourage you to work with essential oils, meditate and journal every day. Make it a joyful self-nurturing ritual. Your psyche will be grateful that you are listening and reward you with more and more insights. This commitment is really at the center of following the path of the Wounded Healer and living our personal myth.

The Practice

1. ***Select an essential oil you want to work with.*** After some
   practice, as mentioned above, you can work with multiple oils.

2. ***Set aside time and make sure you are in a space where you
   won't be interrupted for the duration of the exercise.***

Go into a meditative state, for example by taking a few falling out
breaths and doing abdominal breathing. Center yourself and feel your
feet and sit-bones touching the ground or chair you are in. In this
exercise we will be observing from your heart awareness. You can go
into your heart awareness by tuning in to your heart and opening your
heart doorway. You can switch off your mind, or if that is challenging,
spend some time focusing your mind on observing your breath.

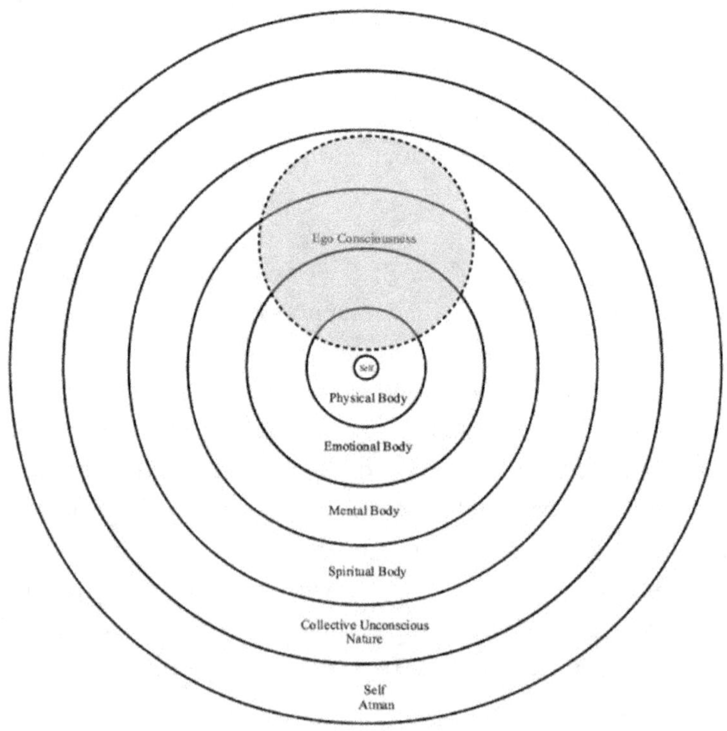

3. *Tune into your Physical Body.*

Essential Oils that can help us tune into the physical body are Vetiver (aka Ruh Khus) (*Vetiveria zizanioides*), Patchouli (*Pogostemon cablin*) & Mitti Attar (*Lutum* in *Santalum album*).

Allow the aroma of the essential oil to enter your physical body. It enters through your airway and goes not just to your lungs but to every part of your body. Feel and observe where in your physical body the aroma goes and where your attention is drawn. If your attention is drawn to an area of your physical body that is uncomfortable, e.g. pain or an illness, merely observe it with your heart awareness. There is no need to judge or try to change or fix what you are being made aware of. Simply acknowledge it and keep your heart awareness open. If your mind tries to take over by focusing on a worry or specific area of your physical body, simply focus your mind on observing your breath and go back into your heart awareness. After one or more areas of your body have come to your attention, open your heart awareness to the parts of your physical body that may have avoided trying to be noticed so far. They may be 'hiding in the background' or you may notice darkness or fog or numbness in certain areas. Allow your heart awareness to notice those, too. It may be helpful to do a body scan, starting from your toes and going up each part of your body to tune in.

Ask yourself:

How did my physical body experience the day?
How embodied or dissociated was I today?
What did my physical body enjoy?
What was challenging for my physical body?
What is my physical body saying to me and asking from me?

4.   *When you are ready, tune into your Emotional Body.*

Essential Oils that can help us tune into the emotional body are
Jasmine Attar (*Jasminium sambac* in *Santalum album*), Rose Attar (*Rosa
damascena* in *Santalum album*) & Ginger Lily Root (aka Kapoor Kachri)
(*Hedychium spicatum*).

If you have difficulty imagining your emotional body, try feeling it as
an invisible body that surrounds your physical body and is a little bit
larger and less dense than your physical body.

Allow the aroma of the essential oil to move through your emotional
body. Feel and observe where in your emotional body the aroma goes
and where your attention is drawn. If your attention is drawn to an
emotion that is uncomfortable, merely observe it with your heart
awareness. There is no need to judge or try to change or fix what you
are being made aware of. Simply acknowledge it and keep your heart
awareness open. If your mind tries to take over by focusing on a
worry or other specific emotion, simply focus your mind on observing
your breath and go back into your heart awareness. After one or more
emotions and areas of your emotional body have come to your
attention, open your heart awareness to the more hidden emotions.
Those are the parts of your emotional body that have not wanted to
be noticed so far. They may be 'hiding in the background' or you may
notice darkness or fog or numbness in certain areas. Allow your heart
awareness to notice those, too.

Ask yourself:

How did my emotional body experience the day?
What emotions were at the forefront today?
How did I process these emotions?
What was challenging emotionally?
What emotions was I unaware of that I was feeling today?
What is my emotional body saying to me and asking me?

5.   *When you are ready, tune into your Mental Body.*

Essential Oils that can help us tune into the mental body are
Rosemary (*Rosmarinus officinalis*), Jasmine essential oil (aka Ruh Bela)
(*Jasminium sambac*) & Galbanum absolute (*Ferula gummosa*).

If you have difficulty imagining your mental body, try feeling it as an
invisible body that surrounds your physical and emotional bodies and
is a little bit larger, invisible and less dense than both your physical
and emotional bodies. You could also imagine it as a river of
thoughts. Usually, we are swept along in the river of our thoughts, but
now imagine you are sitting by the banks of the river, watching the
thoughts go by.

Allow the aroma of the essential oil to move through your mental
body. Feel and observe where in your mental body the aroma goes
and where your attention is drawn. If your attention is drawn to a
thought that is uncomfortable, merely observe it with your heart
awareness. There is no need to judge or try to change or fix what you
are being made aware of, simply acknowledge it and keep your heart
awareness open. If your mind tries to take over by focusing on a
specific thought, simply focus your mind on observing your breath
and go back into your heart awareness. After one or more thoughts
and areas of your mental body have come to your attention, open
your heart awareness to the thoughts and parts of your mental body
that may have avoided noticing so far. They may be 'hiding in the
background' or you may be aware of darkness, fog or numbness in
certain areas. Allow your heart awareness to notice those, too.

Ask yourself:

How did my mental body experience the day?
What thoughts dominated today?
How was my mental body helpful today?
How was it challenging today?
What habitual mental patterns took over today?
What is my mental body saying to me and asking me today?

6. *When you are ready tune into your Spiritual Body.*

Essential Oils that can help us tune into the spiritual body are Sandalwood (*Santalum album*), angelica (root and/or seed) (*Angelica archangelica*) & Tuberose Attar (*Polianthes tuberosa* in *Santalum album*)

If you have difficulty imagining your spiritual body, try feeling it as an invisible body that surrounds your physical, emotional and mental bodies and is a little bit larger, invisible and less dense than those bodies. You could also imagine it as a landscape, since it sits at the interface between the individual and collective unconscious. Even if you don't think you have a spiritual body or a spiritual belief system, you can still tune into this body. It just means it's completely in your unconscious. (I use the word image below, because the content of the spiritual body is more than emotions or thoughts and the word image comes from the Greek word 'imago' meaning cocoon. I use it in this sense of a numinous thought/feeling/sensation that is a cocoon for spirit, instead of the limited sense of image as a picture.)

Allow the aroma of the essential oil to move through your spiritual body. Feel and observe where in your spiritual body the aroma goes and where your attention is drawn. If your attention is drawn to an image or idea that is uncomfortable, merely observe it with your heart awareness. There is no need to judge or try to change or fix what you are being made aware of. Simply acknowledge it and keep your heart awareness open. If your mind tries to take over by focusing on a specific image, simply focus your mind on observing your breath and go back into your heart awareness. After one or more images and areas of your spiritual body have come to your attention, open your heart awareness to the images and parts of your mental body that may have avoided trying to be noticed so far. They may be 'hiding in the background' or you may notice darkness or fog or numbness in certain areas. Allow your heart awareness to notice those, too.

Ask yourself:

How did my spiritual body experience the day?
What unconscious aspect of my spiritual body did I project onto others today?
What was challenging for my spiritual body today?
What is my spiritual body asking of me today?

7. *Tune into the Collective Unconscious.*

This is your rootedness in the world, your family, your ancestors, the parts of Nature that are close to you. Essential Oils that can help us tune into the collective unconscious are Labdanum (*Cistus ladanifer*), Galbanum (*Ferula gummosa*) & Carrot Seed (*Daucus carota*).

Ask yourself:

Did my allies or ancestors connect with me today?
Did I have a strong reaction about anything today?
Did I dream last night and if so, what was the dream about?
What in the collective unconscious can be revealed to me today?
Did any archetypes play out in my life today?
Did I feel any collective energy or emotions today?

8. *Tune into your Self.*

Your Self, called Atman in Sanskrit, is the entirety of every other layer you have tuned in to so far. We glimpse it in moments of awe, when we see how everything is connected and how we (our ego) is just a part. We need to allow our awareness to realize that all the unconscious parts we have just tuned in to are part of ourselves, beyond the ego. The ego may resist this, and try to convince us we are just our ego, but we are so much more than our ego. When we realize we are more than our ego, we are all the other bodies described above, this is a prerequisite for having a glimpse of the Self (with a capital 'S'). The alchemical term for this is Conjunctio, which means marriage. It is the marriage between our conscious ego and the much larger part of us that is our unconscious. In a marriage, neither dominates, so in this case, neither the ego nor the unconscious should dominate. The ego will get messages from the unconscious. Small amounts are gradually made conscious.

Essential Oils that can help us tune into the Self are Champaca (*Magnolia champaca*) and Rose Attar (*Rosa damascena* in *Santalum album*)

Having become aware of all the bodies you've been unconscious of, allow yourself to own all of it and get a sense of your Self, who you truly are, combining ego and unconscious. Feel the energy of this awareness fill you up and ask yourself:

What am I grateful for today?
What is my Self (Atman) wanting me to understand?
What are my Self-intentions for tomorrow?

9. *After you have opened your awareness to each layer of your psyche, slowly come back into your everyday awareness.*

Consider journaling about what themes came up and explore the relationships between themes that came up in the different bodies. You could also make a drawing or a collage. Each time you work with an essential oil, different themes may come to light.

This exercise is helpful in getting into the habit of paying attention to all parts of our psyche, which is useful for working with essential oils as allies, both by themselves and in the context of ketamine and other psychedelic therapy.

Rose Attar

When to use Rose Attar with ketamine or in other psychedelic therapy:

The client needs:
Self-compassion
Self-love
Opening of the heart
To feel loved unconditionally
To feel a spiritual hug
To heal abandonment issues
To heal lack of adequate mothering in childhood

Suggested intentions for using Rose Attar with ketamine or in other psychedelic therapy:

"I want to tune into my heart awareness."
"I want to open my heart."
"I open myself to the loving embrace of rose attar."
"I want to let go of my racing mind and feel my heart awareness."
"I want to feel loved and nurtured."

As mentioned earlier, Rose Attar (*Rosa damascena* in *Santalum album*) is made from the precious, ancient roses cultivated in the Ganges valley near Kannauj. Rose petals (*Rosa spp.*) are hydrodistilled in copper stills and the distillate is captured in sandalwood essential oil. Rose Attar opens the heart. It's like a spiritual hug. It's great for reconnecting to our soul, receiving compassion and feeling self-compassion. I often use this first with clients new to ketamine, if they are nervous about the effects of ketamine. It is also a great support when someone is struggling to tune in to their heart, or remain open hearted, often because of anxiety, both with ketamine and in other psychedelic therapy. I also often use it in combination with other aromas, to provide a sense of being enveloped by love and compassion as the client explores their shadow issues more deeply during the ketamine or other psychedelic experience.

Rose Attar and Opening the Heart Doorway

"The hidden face of nature can only be seen with the heart." –Stephen Harrod Buhner

The heart isn't just a muscle that acts as a pump for the circulatory system. It is also an organ of awareness and perception. When people talk about the heart chakra, this is what they refer to, not just the pump. We can see the world from our brain-mind, yet also from our heart awareness and they are quite different. Our heart can be closed or open, which is language we are all familiar with. Because of this, it is helpful to view the heart as being a doorway that allows for a different way of connecting with everything around us.

When it is opened, the Heart Doorway is the portal for soul-to-soul communication. When we enter the world through the Heart Doorway, we are in the moment, flowing in the knowledge of perception. We only need to pay attention to our connection with the universe, nothing else. Our ego personality takes a back seat and remains passive.

The heart is the bridge between our connection to the sky and spirit and being grounded on earth, in our body. It is the main doorway of perception, while the sky and earth are points of anchorage and stability. It is only with the heart that we can truly learn to receive--to touch and be touched, not just emitting but also receiving information and soulful attention from the world. It is only when we open our heart, that we truly feel the aliveness of the world, in which plants are beings that choose to interact with us. People report that ketamine and other psychedelic therapy makes them feel more connected to everything around them, and the term 'ecodelic' (meaning fostering a deeper sense of connection of the more than human world) has been proposed for this. Being aware of and tuning in to the Heart Doorway and practicing this repeatedly is a foundation for this increased connectedness and ecodelic experience.

Exercise: Bringing Attention to the Heart Doorway

I love Rose Attar for Heart Doorway work, but Melissa (*Melissa officinalis*), Lavender (*Lavandula angustifolia*), Neroli (*Citrus aurantium ssp. amara*) and Rose Geranium (*Pelargonium graveolens*) also have an affinity with the heart.

Sitting comfortably, close your eyes and start to slow down and concentrate on your breath. Follow each breath as you inhale and exhale. If your thoughts wander to other things just bring them back gently to the breath again. When you feel that you are centered and quiet inside and your mind has stopped chatting and distracting you, bring your attention to the Heart Center. When I do this, I always feel a flutter in my heart as my attention activates it. For some people this area can initially feel closed and cold. This is not a problem. It just means that this exercise is an important one for you and one that you will need to practice often. It is like any form of exercise. If we haven't used a certain muscle or set of muscles, they become stiff and weak and need regular gentle exercise to open. It is the same for opening the Heart Doorway.

Imagine a beautiful rose opening in the Heart Center, each and every petal reaching outwards expansively. Continue to breathe and focus your attention on the opening rose. You may feel the subtle sensation of an opening movement.

Vetiver (Ruh Khus)

When to use Vetiver (Ruh Khus) with ketamine and other psychedelic therapy:

The client:
Needs grounding, both in life and during the ketamine experience.
Is ready to leave dissociation behind.
Is ready to be more fully embodied.

Suggested intentions for using Vetiver with ketamine:

"I am ready to feel grounded and in my body."
"I am ready to leave the fortress of my mind/intellect and connect
with the other parts of myself."

There are many grounding oils, but not all of them have Vetiver's safe
and earthy quality. Ruh Khus is the Hindi name for wild Vetiver.
Vetiver *(Vetiveria zizanioides)* has a deeply earthy pulse with a slightly
smoky note, which then leads into a smell of texture—The texture of
embodiment, grounded reality and dried, cut wood.

In 'Aromatherapy for Healing the Spirit' Gabriel Mojay describes
vetiver as being *'…imbued with the calm, reassuring strength of mother earth'*
and this really sums it up. It helps us to be grounded and connected
to the earth, which is really important for being wholly embodied in a
softly powerful way. Vetiver *'centers and reconnects us.'*

Vetiver encourages us let go of using the intellect as our armor or
castle and to really feel at home in our bodies and discover what it
feels like to be fully alive and present in our physical bodies. If we are

prone to dissociation, vetiver grounds us. In brief, grounding can be defined as the opposite of dissociation. For people who are chronically dissociated, the grounding and embodying experience that Vetiver offers can be very unusual. You could almost say that for them, being embodied is a Non-Ordinary State of Consciousness (NOSC), which ketamine and other psychedelic therapy can allow, when it is not accessible to habitual ego consciousness.

By building a solid, loving relationship with our physical bodies, we begin to feel more confident and centered. Our feelings, thoughts, emotions and interactions are anchored in our flesh and bones.

All the energy of Vetiver is in its roots, which are deeply penetrating. It is cultivated along riverbanks to reinforce the earth and avoid soil erosion. It does the same for humans. Its energy helps us descend into our root chakra, bringing us into our body and safety.

This oil helps us to inhabit our physical bodies and to live in them fully. It can help us remember our ancestral roots and connect with our own original material. It reminds us of our inner temple while at the same time being very appeasing and comforting for the mind. By re-connecting deeply with our physical bodies—our inner earth—we find a feeling of confidence in ourselves and in life.

Another use of Vetiver can be to ground people back in their body when the ketamine or psychedelic therapy have made them feel very disconnected from their body, or that they even have no body. If someone is struggling with this, having them smell Vetiver and also Yarrow essential oil can bring them back into their body powerfully and rapidly. Yarrow is very good for helping form boundaries, so you could think of it as having the opposite effect of ketamine and psychedelic therapy, which help dissolve ego boundaries. Other than this particular indication, to help someone come back into their body, I wouldn't use yarrow essential oil with ketamine or other psychedelic therapy.

Grounding Exercise

I find this exercise is really helpful regardless of where I am and especially helpful during times when it's easy to be stuck in unconscious patterns—Stuck in an airplane seat, waiting at a traffic light, rushing from place to place. It's great to practice with clients before they experience ketamine or other psychedelic therapy.

Close your eyes halfway, even briefly if you can. Smell Vetiver (ruh khus).

Take a few falling out breaths, inhaling deeply through your nose and exhaling all the stress and distractedness deeply through your mouth.

Then try to observe your breathing, not forcing it, but just observing as your body is moved by the tide of air in and out. Remember that this air is what connects all living beings. We are all breathing the same air and it is the invisible presence between us all.

As you observe your breath and the air moving in and out, with your awareness, direct your breath deeper and deeper into your abdomen, your inner soil, your belly button.

After a few breaths, when you feel you've connected through awareness to your abdomen, direct your breath with your awareness all the way to the bottom of your feet. See if you can be aware of the invisible rainbows at the bottom of your feet.

When you feel fully connected to your abdomen and your feet, from the perspective of your body, connect to your busy mind and reconnect it to your groundedness. As your awareness now moves upward, remember that your awareness resides in your heart and your heart connects all the parts of your being and connects you to the beings around you and spirit.

Once you have connected feet, abdomen, busy mind and heart, through the heart doorway, connect to nature around you—a tree, or plants nearby. If you're somewhere where it feels like there's no plants nearby, open yourself to their presence. It might be a potted plant, a weed surviving in a sidewalk crack or a tree nearby. If you really can't connect with a plant around you, take your awareness to a strong memory of spending time with your favorite tree or plant or a place in Nature, or a time when you really felt connected to Nature.

Try to do this for as long as you can, even if it's just a few moments while stuck in traffic. Ideally set aside time in nature and really savor the connectedness.

Galbanum

When to use Galbanum with ketamine and psychedelic therapy:

The client:
Struggles to commit to or manifest changes in their life.
Is struggling with making excuses and lack of focus.
Is afraid of what ketamine may bring up that is ready to be processed.
Would benefit from connecting with their ancestral strength

Suggested intentions for using Galbanum with ketamine:

"I am ready to commit to the path forward and to changing these specific thoughts and behaviors."
"I am ready to face myself and to discover my inner strength."

Galbanum absolute is made from the resin of a Persian species of fennel called *Ferula gummosa*. In the old testament, it's mentioned as one of the ingredients in Ketoret, the sacred Jewish incense that's burned on the Sabbath. One of its purposes is to carry the sacred energy of the sabbath into the other days of the week.

I have found galbanum essential oil to be a great aroma for committing to change and a new path, e.g. for helping clients with addiction commit to sobriety. It is great for helping us to stop delaying and waiting around and take action and commit to the path ahead. 'The time is now,' it seems to say. In combination with ketamine, it appears to really help committing to the changes the neuroplasticity of ketamine offers, but which require changes in behavior and thought patterns.

It is also powerful in bringing up Shadow issues and allowing the client to go more deeply into the ketamine experience to retrieve insights that are ready to be released from the unconscious into consciousness, but that the ego may be resisting out of fear of change.

Galbanum is a powerful ally, that forces us to believe and to carry on, and to do all the necessary work. Galbanum gives us inner strength, pushing us to action. It supports us during the challenges of surviving and healing. It helps us be a strong enough vessel for the deep, fiery, uncontrollable emotions that burst through and allows us to break down and allow more of our authentic selves to surface. It reminds us to stop looking outwards and dive inwards.

Galbanum is a teacher that is great for pilgrimages (both inner and outer), for helping us fully commit to our path, even and especially when we don't glimpse the still hidden goal or center or the meaning which reveals itself slowly step by step.

Galbanum has a very masculine energy, strong and forthright, no beating around the bush. It makes us feel that it believes in us, confident that we can be ourselves, confident that we can hold all the feelings that need to be acknowledged, that have been hiding for so long. It brings a focus to the healing and invites the allies and ancestors in. Galbanum is a guardian of the work that has yet to be done. When we are on the threshold, it makes sure everything is in the right place for deep healing. Galbanum is a warrior of the heart and doesn't want excuses or time-wasting. Galbanum knows we can do it and reminds us of the motivation, the energy behind the action. With galbanum we can re-write our personal myth.

Labdanum

When to use Labdanum with ketamine and psychedelic therapy:

The client:
Is ready to face what is waiting to be brought up from the Shadow
into ego consciousness, including the hidden gifts of traumas or other
challenging experiences.
Has repressed traumas or other important memories that they are
ready to remember.

Suggested intentions for using Labdanum with ketamine:

"I am ready to see what is waiting to come up from the Shadow."
"I am ready to understand the hidden gift of the trauma(s) I
experienced."
"I am ready to embrace the power that has been hiding in my
Shadow."

Labdanum is the aromatic resin of the cistus shrub (*Cistus ladanifer*)
and one of the oldest known aromatic substances. The resin secreted
by the cistus shrub was harvested in ancient times by collecting the
wool of the sheep that grazed among and rubbed against the shrubs.
It was highly revered in ancient times. Egyptian pharaohs rubbed
labdanum in their beards and labdanum is deeply linked with Osiris,
who holds a 'flail', which is really a device for collecting labdanum in
his hand. Osiris was the link between the world of the living and the
dead, which you could think of as shadows of each other. In ancient
Sumeria, warriors rubbed it all over their skin after returning from
battle. Again, there is a clue in this description that it helped warriors
process their experiences and their shadow sides before rejoining
society.

It has a very directive energy, that goes straight to the task and heightens our awareness and consciousness. It helps us unearth hidden aspects of ourselves and our family systems—the individual and collective Shadow. Labdanum sharpens our senses and our sense of spirit. It helps us to focus, not get way laid and not let our energy get dispersed. It helps to liberate traumatic cellular memories that have been repressed and it exposes the lies and silences in unhealthy family systems.

We call this oil *the Master of the Shadow*. It is the most powerful aromatic ally that we know for working with aspects of our ancestral journeys that are hidden but ready to come forward, ready to move up and out from our cellular memory.

This oil is wild and cannot be tamed. It does what it feels is best and goes to the places where it knows there is shadow material waiting to come through. It also opens up our mental bodies, liberates our senses and our spirit, making us very lucid, sharpening our consciousness. This enables us to be very aware of what is going on in our unconscious and to be able to capture the shadow material as it rises from within ourselves. Unknown parts of ourselves start to make themselves known. There is no hanging about, or aimlessly waiting, with this oil. It goes to where it needs to go and will not give up until it has unearthed what needs to be unearthed. It definitely gets the job done. Ancient memories, cellular memories and ancestral memories are loosened by this oil's presence. Family secrets, silences and false family myths are exposed.

Labdanum knows how to reveal what is hidden but ready to be bought into the light. Its wild, earthy, animal aroma is reflected in its energy. You cannot control labdanum. It will cut through the superficial levels to where it needs to go. The key is to trust that it will navigate the shadow realm until what is below the surface can rise. It is very persistent and focused in revealing unknown parts of ourselves. It awakens our instinctual knowing and doesn't allow us to hide from ourselves or disperse our energy. It is able to liberate cellular memories from trauma in childhood, ancestral memories, etc., that have been stored in the body's cells and that are ready to be liberated and made conscious.

In combination with ketamine or other psychedelic therapy, it can be extremely powerful.

Labdanum and the Shadow

Learning to allow shadow elements of ourselves to come into the light and be recognized is a large aspect of the healing journey, as Jung stated when he said, "We become enlightened, not by imagining figures of light but by fearlessly confronting our Shadow." A common mistake people make when thinking about the Shadow is to think that it is made up entirely of 'negative', shameful aspects of ourselves that we are trying to repress. In that view, the Shadow is both what we don't want people to see and things that we're actively trying to suppress. While that is a part of the Shadow, i.e. a part of the personal Shadow, that is in close interaction with the ego to prop up the Persona (our mask to the world), there is another, less personal and more archetypal dimension to the Shadow. It's the rest of the iceberg so to speak.

Our cultures, societies and upbringing play a large role in teaching a child what is acceptable behavior and what is not. We learn very young to suppress those parts of ourselves that are considered undesirable and they become part of our shadow. This is the personal or ego Shadow.

Although the parts of ourselves we see as negative are one aspect of the Shadow, it is not the whole picture. In fact, you could say that if you are conscious of something that you see negatively about yourself, it is no longer in the Shadow, since you are conscious of it. However, we often have unconscious judgements about ourselves.

As an archetype, the Shadow basically encompasses everything that we do not know about ourselves, both positive and negative, including instincts, beliefs and ideas that we have for some reason kept from the light of consciousnesses. Our greatest power and gifts are often hidden in our Shadow. We may have learnt as a child for example that our strength was a threat to adults and other children around us and so we have hidden our strength in the personal Shadow and are unconscious of our own strength. There are hidden treasures in our Shadow. In her poem "Our Greatest Fear", Marianne Williamson says:

It is our light not our darkness that most frightens us
Our deepest fear is not that we are inadequate.
Our deepest fear is that we are powerful beyond measure.
It is our light not our darkness that most frightens us.

The Shadow exists not only on a personal level as described above but there is also a collective Shadow. We see this in the world today and throughout history, when a group of people consider themselves 'pure' and 'right' and 'superior' and project their own Shadow on another group that is considered 'impure', 'wrong' and 'inferior.' This happens unconsciously and on a collective level and is an archetypal force, which is why it can sweep through countries and civilizations quickly and make people seem possessed and act out the worst archetypes unconsciously. Jung, somewhat controversially, felt that this is what happened in Nazi Germany, when the Nazis projected their own darkness onto Jewish people.

The problem with the Shadow is that if we do not recognize it as existing and work on bringing it into the light, it controls us much more powerfully. The main way it manifests is through projection, which is always unconscious. Jung himself said that the most important cultural and political work any of us can do is to own our Shadow projections. What we do not accept as part of ourselves, we tend to unconsciously project onto others. For example, in most cases when we have a strong feeling of hate, obsession or infatuation towards another person, it is usually a sign that we are projecting a part of our Shadow onto them. We can project 'negative' aspects of ourselves unconsciously, when we 'hate' someone, but we can also project our own unconscious power onto someone, e.g. when we feel someone is our 'guru'. Next time this happens to you, stop and take the time to draw back in those strong feelings and see if you can identify some aspect of yourself that you are unconscious of and that is asking to be accepted by your consciousness as part of you. Journaling is a good way of working through these strong feelings and unearthing the hidden treasures the Shadow hides.

When we are able to accept and assimilate our Shadow, we accept ourselves on a deeper level, we can forgive our shortcomings and liberate the creative energy that was blocked in repressing the parts of our Shadow that are ready to be integrated. We stop trying to be perfect and recognize that becoming whole is more important in the journey towards individuation.

It is important to remember that everyone has a Shadow. Where there is light there is undeniably shadow. The Shadow is bottomless, like every archetype. The idea is not to eventually rid ourselves of every aspect of our Shadow, which is impossible, but to be constantly integrating the parts of the Shadow that are nearest to the light and through our projections asking us to acknowledge them. This is one aspect of the *conjunctio*, the alchemical equivalent of 'enlightenment': The sacred marriage between the conscious ego and the unconscious Shadow. Neither must dominate, but each must be honored.

"If you imagine someone who is brave enough to withdraw all his projections, then you get an individual who is conscious of a pretty thick shadow. Such a man has saddled himself with new problems and conflicts. He has become a serious problem to himself, as he is now unable to say that they do this or that, they are wrong, and they must be fought against... Such a man knows that whatever is wrong in the world is in himself, and if he only learns to deal with his own shadow, he has done something real for the world. He has succeeded in shouldering at least an infinitesimal part of the gigantic, unsolved social problems of our day." (C. G.

Jung, "Psychology and Religion" (1938). In CW 11: Psychology and Religion: West and East. P.140)

The Shadow is not only part of the individual unconscious psyche, family and collective shadows also exist. Secrets and traumatic events that have not been allowed to process naturally are held in the genealogical Shadow, both in families and social groups. Because the psychic processes are inevitable, someone will be born into such a genealogical line with a soul pull to reveal and bring this Shadow into the light for healing. These Shadow aspects are held in our cellular memories that get passed down through with DNA, in what has recently been shown by trauma researchers as the epigenetic inheritance of trauma.

On a cultural or collective level, countries and peoples also have a Shadow, the part of themselves they are not willing or capable of seeing and that they may project onto countries or groups. Sometimes the projection is mutual, as between the US and Soviet Union during the Cold War. As Jung said, "the world hangs by a thin thread and that thread is the human psyche."

Exercise: Connecting with our Shadow with labdanum

Make sure that you are comfortable and will not be disturbed. Whilst smelling the labdanum, ask yourself the question, "What needs to be revealed from my shadow?" or "What is ready to come from my shadow into the light?"

Allow the labdanum to do the work. I have found all I need to do is keep the question in mind visualizing my cells opening and releasing tiny bubbles of information. (I see the bubbles like champagne bubbles that rise up from the bottom of a champagne glass). Whilst witnessing the work, try and catch the information that rises. It may come as a word, a feeling or sensation, a visual picture. Remember there is no wrong or right, there is just what is. Once you feel the work is over, use your journal to note down anything that came up.

Helichrysrum

When to use Helichrysum with ketamine or other psychedelic therapy:

The client:
Is unable to cry tears that have long needed to come up.
Needs to heal old, even childhood trauma.
Is ready to heal psychic 'bruises' and wounds.

Suggested intentions for using Helichrysum with ketamine:

"I am ready to feel the tears that are waiting to come."
"I am ready to understand the hidden gift of the trauma(s) I experienced."
"I am ready to embrace the power that has been hiding in my Shadow."

Helichrysum essential oil is made from a Mediterranean shrub (*Helichrysum italicum*) that is also called immortelle or everlasting, because its flowers appear not to wilt. Helichrysum is great for releasing and healing childhood trauma. It allows us to cry long-suppressed tears and facilitates deep release coupled with a feeling self-compassion. You can finally allow yourself to feel without judgement. It also reminds you that it is much healthier to allow these deeply repressed feelings to surface than to be continually running from them. Helichrysum goes to the core, it doesn't beat about the bush. In the context of ketamine, it's great for those who lack self-compassion and need to cry the tears they have never allowed to come up.

Helichrysum oil is an ally for our time, when many of us are reeling in shock, sadness, fear and even despair at the state of our world. We are definitely dealing with an aspect of humanity and our psyches that needs to be addressed by us all and disarmed. (You can read more about this here: https://cathysattars.com/helichrysum-an-ally-for-challening-times/)

High quality, alive Helichrysum essential oil is rare. The power of the oil comes from the sun and the land. It grows abundantly on extremely deprived, stony earth so that it can help heal the land with the wildlife that are attracted by it and with its powerful solar force.

In the same way as this plant is called to heal the dry, stony land where it grows, I feel it is called to help us heal the parts of ourselves that were hurt or neglected when we were younger or growing up. On smelling it, it immediately touches our deepest self, our essence. Like the sun that it has such a strong affinity with, it lights up, warms and brings to life the deeply hidden self or abandoned inner child.

This amazing oil not only helps the body to reabsorb physical bruises, but it also helps the soul reabsorb the emotional and psychological bruises and shocks of both the present and the past. It is an incredibly, powerful healer for the soul, bringing inner peace and self-compassion to the forefront while strengthening our relationship with the unconscious realms.

Its ability to bring a sense of inner peace makes it a great ally in periods of life that are emotionally, physically and spiritually challenging.

In terms of what is happening in the world today, many of us are feeling a combination of sadness, grief, fear for the future and disbelief. We do not know what to do, how to make a stand, how to help change things. Helichrysum brings a sense of inner conciliation and non-violence that stimulates creative action and brings a clear vision to the best and most authentic way each of us can 'act' in our lives and in this crazy world. I personally am really grateful to have it beside me as an ally and although it took a long time coming, it definitely showed up when it was most needed.

As usual, we recommend that you just smell the oil in order to benefit from its qualities. However, for emotional shocks and traumas you could also put a drop under each foot and on the solar plexus.

Suggested Protocols

There are a number of different approaches to using ketamine for psychedelic therapy. Some therapists work with lower doses and talk with the client during the acute experience. Others use higher doses (which are more dissociative and thus make it difficult to talk during the acute experience) and talk with the client before and after the immediate effects. There are different routes, including intramuscular injection (im), intravenous infusion (iv), sublingual troches, intranasal sprays, and others. Each has their unique duration and effect. In general, im and iv are more powerful and more rapid in onset and shorter in duration. Many therapists also have preparatory sessions before starting ketamine treatments and debriefing/integration sessions after treatment. The use of aromatic allies can be adapted to all of these different settings.

The different approaches and protocols to other forms of psychedelic therapy, such as with psilocybin and MDMA are also varied. At the time of this writing, both of these are still awaiting FDA approval. Even if certain protocols are FDA approved, there are many different approaches, some of which are being formally studied. Other approaches, including those based on traditional indigenous practices, may not be formally studied, but may still offer profound healing. In many of these, incorporating aromas as discussed here with an emphasis on ketamine, offers an opportunity for the person undergoing therapy and for the practitioner to have deeper, more heart-felt and transformative experiences, because aromas bypass the intellect and touch all aspects of the psyche, as discussed above. Especially when practiced beforehand, during preparation sessions, they can give the person a sense of being a more active participant in the experience by smelling aromas.

In the context of larger doses of ketamine as well as other psychedelic therapies, psychedelic research has confirmed that the likelihood of a negative experience (a 'bad trip') can be minimized by having a clear intention and having experienced sitters during the experience. In the setting of higher dosage treatments, because the ketamine experience can be intense, inward and dissociative, a sitter isn't commonly able to talk to the client during the experience. Some clients like to have a trusted friend or family member be present in lieu of a sitter and in those cases this person should be instructed on the basics of being a good sitter, i.e. being non-directive, avoiding anxiety or other negative emotions and holding the space with a neutral, open, benevolent attitude.

How to use the oils with ketamine and other psychedelic therapies

The easiest way to work with aromas is to use the scent strips, also known as perfume test strips. You can dip the scent strip in the bottle or put a drop of the oil at one end of the scent strip. That way gives you and the client the most control. You can put the scent strip near the client's face, e.g. on their chest if they are lying back in a recliner and if they client doesn't like the smell they can take the scent strip and remove it. During im or iv ketamine, since the experience is so brief, usually the client only needs to work with one or at most two aromas. With longer duration forms of ketamine (sublingual, intranasal, other) and other forms of psychedelic therapy, over the course of time, you may present the client with a number of aromas.

I don't recommend the use of diffusers for several reasons. One is that most diffusers, that work by heat or use water, change the chemistry of the essential oils, in the worst case even burning them. Even if that is not a problem, when you use a diffuser, you fill the entire room with the aroma, which can be overwhelming to you and the client and makes it difficult to get rid of an aroma or introduce new aromas. If you use the same space for several ketamine sessions in the same day, for example, it is very difficult to remove all the aroma in the room that has been filled by a diffuser between clients.

With regards to selecting an aroma, you can discuss the various properties of the aromatic allies and suggest an oil based on the client's issues or intentions. This is also based on your familiarity with the aromas, which you get by smelling them and working with them repeatedly, especially by themselves, i.e. not as part of psychedelic therapy.

You can also let the client smell the oils, or a selection of oils you think appropriate, and select an oil based on the client's reaction to the smell. When judging the client's reaction, pay attention to your own intuition as you present the particular oil. Also look at the client's face, as their face may express something different than their words. You may notice the client smiling or having an open face, but they may say 'I'm not sure' or 'that's an unusual smell' or even 'I don't like it.' Use all the information, i.e. your intuition, the client's expression and their words to select the oil. As you work with the oils and they become your allies, your intuition and judgement will deepen.

Once you and the client have selected an oil, dip the pointed end of the scent strip in the vial. You can give the client a scent strip and smell the bottle yourself or you can use two scent strips (one for the client, one for you.)

In general, we recommend starting with one aroma at a time. As you gain more experience, you can experiment with combining two aromas. Remember that each aroma is the manifestation of a living plant spirit and each aroma can teach us a lot of different things.

Using Aromatic Allies in Preparation Sessions
(before Ketamine or other psychedelic therapy)

Using one of the aromas in the kit, you could guide the client through
the Concentric Circles discussed earlier so they have a more thorough
and complete sense of the issues that may be ready to be transformed
in their psyche or at least get a better sense of the hidden areas that
could be explored deeper in the ketamine experience.

You can also discuss the client's intention while smelling one of the
aromas. When the client then smells the aroma during the ketamine
experience, this may allow the intention to be brought into the
experience through the associative power of aroma.

Using Aromatic Allies During the Experience

Decide on one aroma together with the client. Give the client a scent
strip. It may be easiest to have the client hold it in one hand, so they
can bring it closer to their nose or remove it as needed. If you use two
aromas, put one in each hand, since any more than that can be
confusing and overwhelming during higher dose ketamine sessions
due to the dissociative effects of ketamine. Alternatively, if the client
is in a recliner, they could put the scent strip on their chest in front of
their face. If you use ketamine in lower doses, the client may be more
easily able to hold scent strips and interact with you and you could
present the clients with different scent strips during the session.
You can use a similar technique for other psychedelic therapies.
Consider that, because of the longer duration, you may offer multiple
aromas to the client during their experience, using one or at most two
aromas at a time.

Using Aromatic Allies after a Ketamine or Other Psychedelic Session

In a follow up session, you can revisit the aroma or aromas you used to see if they allow the client to access the insights gained during the ketamine or other psychedelic experience. You could go through the Concentric Circles again and see how the inner landscape of the psyche has changed. In order to continue to access the insights, you could give the client a small vial with a few drops of the aroma or aromas used, so they can smell them throughout the day to help with integrating their insights and remembering their intentions. (You can buy small vials, e.g. 1ml, online easily. They are the size of perfume sample vials.) The client could also use the aroma to smell while journaling (automatic writing) or making art (drawing, collage, etc.) to continue to deepen the communication between the ego and the unconscious.

Because this is an emerging and developing field, the above suggestions are just that--suggestions. You can adapt the use of aromas to your unique practice and the needs of your clients. Remember, as mentioned earlier, that MDMA, which may become FDA approved soon, appears to dull the sense of scent. Even without a conscious sense of scent, our bodies react to aromas, but the best way to use aromas with MDMA is worth of exploration.

Also, don't forget that you can use aromas by themselves, without psychedelic therapy, and thus the aromas can become a daily practice and everyday allies for you and your clients on your journeys of individuation.

Addendum: The Compassionate Void

When we experience ketamine and sometimes other psychedelics, some of us have the experience of entering a void. With ketamine some people refer to this as the 'k-hole.' Another term is ego-death. In the context of trauma-spectrum disorders and PTSD, extreme dissociation can feel like entering this void. The recent movie 'Get Out', which deals with the deep trauma of racism called this experience 'the sunken place.' It can be a challenging or overwhelming experience, but I have come to realize that this void is compassionate and want to share my experience of it. Perhaps you or your clients find it helpful in navigating and making friends with the Void.

The awareness or the feeling that the Void is compassionate first came to me during a psychic journey several years ago. I had visited the Void many times before since early childhood, in dissociation due to trauma and emotional neglect. It was a scary place to go for many years, when involuntarily pushed there by trauma and triggers, causing a feeling of total ego dissolution, no way to navigate and feeling stuck there, no way out. The image I had was that I was a disembodied thing floating in infinite darkness over an endless cold concrete surface. I didn't have any residual awareness, or more precisely heart awareness, that allowed me to recognize it and navigate it.

The way to recognize it is to feel it, using our heart awareness. If we go into the Void with this awareness and using aromatic allies, they can take us there, guide us through it, make the feelings more real and intense and at the same time help us maintain our heart awareness. Instead of feeling stuck, with no way out, we can receive the wisdom of the Void. It was during one of these journeys with essential oils and plant spirit medicine that I overwhelmingly felt and directly experienced that the Void was compassionate.

I couldn't make sense of my own experience of the Void being compassionate, I just felt it, until I read about the relationship between the Tibetan buddhist 'deities' Avalokitesvara (The 1000-armed Bodhisattva of Compassion) and Mahakala (The Great Black One, personification of the Void) and that they are two manifestations of the same archetype. Archetypes always constellate as seeming paradoxes, or pairs of opposites. Mahakala is the shadow of Avalokitesvara and vice versa.

This paradoxical quality of an archetype is symbolized in descriptions of the alchemical philosopher's stone, which is the goal of the alchemical quest and archetypal symbol of the Self. In ancient alchemical texts, the philosopher's stone is described as both 'dead and alive', 'masculine and feminine', 'black and white', 'hot and cold'. There are countless other examples. These paradoxes point at some deeper truth that is beyond language. The only term I find comes close is 'numinous' which means 'having a strong religious or spiritual quality; indicating or suggesting the presence of a divinity.' To me numinous is a word that hints at that sacred feeling we get, the awe and goosebumps when we have glimpses of the higher perspective from which the paradoxes are resolved. I think this is most poetically expressed in 1 Corinthians 13:12 (NIV): "For now we see only a reflection as in a mirror; then we shall see face to face. Now I know in part; then I shall know fully, even as I am fully known."

Similarly, there's an archetype of which Avalokitesvara is the benevolent, 'nice', 'light' manifestation and Mahakala the 'malevolent', 'Dark' manifestation. They seem like opposites of each other, e.g. Mahakala is usually represented black and Avalokitesvara white; Mahakala seemingly wrathful in a terrifying dancing stance, Avalokitesvara sitting blissfully. Yet at the root, they are the same. So, when we encounter Mahakala, the terrifying Void, if we remember this, we can maintain some awareness greater than our ego while the Void takes us. Then as we travel into the Void, and all the negative feelings, beliefs and thoughts come up, like the headlights of a car in a night storm, we can see a little bit ahead of us. We can't see the whole way, but even if we just see a little bit ahead, like the car, we eventually get there. Fear, self-recrimination and other challenging emotions that may come up are the gatekeepers so to say, like the sphinx at the entrance to Thebes or the Fu Dogs outside Chinese temples. Those fears and negative thoughts, as intense and distracting and awareness-dissolving as they are, are a sign that we are moving in the right direction. Remembering that helps us a little further along. While it feels like we may be overtaken by Mahakala or his realm, at some point, like night turning into dawn, this experience will transform and you feel this compassion, the gift of Avalokitesvara.

Through the journey through the Void you'll get a visceral feeling for what I can only describe in a limited way with words now. The self-recrimination and the fears, and the self-love, self-awe and commitment to the path of individuation are flipsides of the same coin. You will go through the alchemical process, reconciling the opposites and see things from a higher, different perspective.

When you encounter your fear and self-recrimination, it helps to imagine it as some sort of personification, a person or an animal or imaginary being. And you can ask it what it wants and needs, and you can send it love. This is a very nutshell description of a Tibetan Buddhist practice called Choed, which is a powerful framework for encountering parts of ourselves that terrify us, i.e. our Shadow.

Some of us or our clients may feel we don't really know how to keep traveling far inside of us, into the void. It can feel like an endless slog. It may feel there's just more trauma and misery to uncover and no clear 'payoff'. The alchemical literature is full of stories of alchemists who 'wandered in the desert for years', which to me metaphorically describes the same process.

What keeps motivating me is that if we don't answer the call of our Soul when it calls us, the alternatives are insanity or death. Jung, in his mythobiography 'Memories, Dreams, Reflections' talks about a client who refused to go into his own depth when his soul was calling and became obsessed with mountain climbing, wanting to higher and higher in the outside world to avoid going deeper within himself. The client died in a mountain climbing accident and Jung felt he had committed 'spiritual suicide.' His soul only gave him so many chances and when he refused and avoided, his Soul said, 'Game Over'. Following our Soul, into the void if necessary is difficult path, but it's the 'only' path forward. And the alchemical model reminds us that we can transform these unconscious energies, feelings, thought patterns into stepping-stones for growth.

That new perspective has been called the Alchemical third (often pictured as a divine child in alchemical illustrations such as the series of woodcuts called the 'rosa philosophorum'). Jung called it the '10,000-year-old man.' The 10,000-year-old man is within us, but in our imagination appears to us quite different from our ego and we need to transcend the boundaries and limitations of the ego to viscerally feel this other level of awareness, this new perspective.

Being beheld, truly beheld by another, is very helpful for 'holding the space', the awareness, that allows us to tolerate this process. But we can't be with someone to behold us all the time. In a way this being beheld is the true healing of a deep therapy session, with or without psychedelics. The essence of healing is beholding. The beholding in a therapy session is really only practice for developing the capacity to behold ourselves. It doesn't make it any easier, the energy just gets more intense. The tantric deities that are sitting on fire or in the sexual act represent the intensity of this process. As you continue to explore the unconscious realms, you can ask for guides on the 'other side', i.e.

in the psychic realm. At first it could be a plant or animal ally, a psychopomp, then it can be that personification of our wisdom, and then outside the personal unconscious, we encounter the ancestors. You can call on any of these to be by your side when you're journeying there.

This process is scary and it's easy to distract ourselves with mundane tasks in the material world, and focusing on other people, but if we do it mindfully, i.e. to recharge our batteries between psychic journeys it can be very grounding. This is to me the deeper meaning of the old story 'chop wood, carry water.' We need to be grounded in our body and the material world, especially Nature, so we can safely travel into the infinite void inside ourselves.

Godspeed.

Additional Resources

To order the essential oils discussed, please visit *cathysattars.com*

I have created a kit of 5 essential oils called the Psychedelic Therapy Support kit, which you can order from cathysattars.com: *https://cathysattars.com/product/psychedelic-therapy-support-kit/*

I have created a more in-depth, self-paced online class, which will give you a lot more information:

https://aromagnosis.com/essential-oils-for-psychedelic-therapy/

To learn more about our approach, read our blogs and subscribe to our newsletters. Each of our websites, *cathysattars.com* and *aromagnosis.com* have a separate blog and newsletter. You can sign up for the newsletters on each of the sites.

We also have a YouTube channel in which we discuss our approach:

https://tinyurl.com/aromagnosisyoutube

If you are interested in a consultation with us, visit
https://aromagnosis.com/individual-consultations-with-cathy-and-florian/

About the Authors

Florian Birkmayer, MD My calling is to help people find their soul's purpose in collaboration with my wife Cathy Skipper. We use aromatics in the form of essential oils, the expressions of the plants' souls, because they are powerful living allies to heal the relationship between the different parts of ourselves, so that these parts cooperate instead of clashing. Through my commitment to my own Wounded Healer's journey, I share with our clients and students my deep understanding of what it is to be human and find your own personal myth or soul's purpose.

After a career in mainstream academic psychiatry and addiction treatment, I became frustrated by the overemphasis on pharmaceuticals to cover up symptoms and decided to use my knowledge and experience to help people recover from pharmaceutical medications. I received my bachelor's degree in molecular biology at Princeton University, where I learned to question assumptions and discover the hidden gifts of the unseen side of life, the shadow. I received my medical doctorate from Columbia University, which taught me how to think critically about 'business-as-usual' medicine and inspired me to become an addiction psychiatrist, since I felt that all physical disease has its origins in imbalances in the psyche, especially trauma, an idea which had been shunned by most of medicine. I know viscerally that our life's challenges, such as traumas, can be turned into steppingstones on the path of our personal myth and living our soul's purpose.

Selected Publications

Birkmayer F. (2022). Essential Oils for the Wounded Healer: PTSD, Post-Traumatic Resilience and the Wounded Healer's Journey. International Journal of Professional Holistic Aromatherapy. 11(3), p. 37-41.

Birkmayer F. (2021). Using Essential Oils to Enhance the Effects of Ketamine Psychedelic Therapy in Obsessive Compulsive Disorder and Substance-Induced Psychosis (Two Case Reports). International Journal of Professional Holistic Aromatherapy. 9(4), p.15-22.

Birkmayer F. (2020). The Molecules of Connectedness. International Journal of Professional Holistic Aromatherapy. 8(4), p. 51-57.

Birkmayer F., Skipper C. (2018). "The Role of Aromatherapy in the Treatment of Substance Abuse and Co-Occurring Disorders", chapter in Modir S. & Munuz G. (eds.) Integrative Addiction and Recovery, Weil Integrative Medicine Library, Oxford University Press, ISBN 9780190275334

Cathy Skipper began her career in the healing arts. She trained at The Royal Central School of Speech and Drama where she studied Drama, Applied Theater and Education. She worked in schools and social settings using drama as the medium for healing. Cathy moved to rural France in her mid-twenties and learnt to live in nature, travelling with a horse and cart and living off the land. In 2003, she settled in the South-East of France farming blueberries, medicinal plants and making organic wine. At the same time, she trained at Ecole Lyonnaise de Plantes. She went on to teach field botany, practical herbalism, gardening and aromatherapy at the school as well as coauthoring an aromatherapy book with the director of the school, Patrice de Bonneval. In 2014, Cathy met her husband Florian Birkmayer, MD and since then they have founded their own school called, AromaGnosis. which combines aromatherapy, psychology, plant consciousness, spirituality and personal journeying for healing the whole person. Cathy wrote the book and online class "The Alchemy of Menopause" in 2018 and is currently writing a new book on 'Decolonizing the Motherline."